Getting the Real Secrets of an Essential Oil

A Complete Guide on Natural Remedies
with Essential Oil Recipes!

By

Angel Burns

License Notices

Table of Contents

Introduction

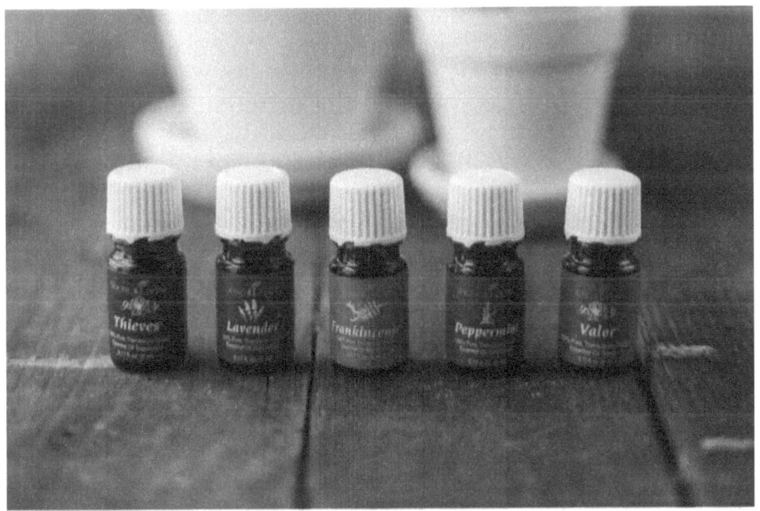

Welcome to the beauty of aromatherapy! Essential oils can be used for cooking, for household, for beauty products. Whatever you need, they can surely perform and deliver.

Essential Oils are key to living a healthy life that is not only sustainable, but also effective. The large amount of chemicals that companies put into our makeup, lotions, and skincare products has caused many people to move toward essential oils, making it such a burgeoning field.

This book will demonstrate to you what you need to know to get started using essential oils. I'll be discussing the different types of essential oils and all of their amazing benefits to our health and healing. I'll also be going over a ton of easy to create essential oil recipes and the different ways they can be used to improve your life. I hope you will fall in love with essential oils the same way I have over the years.

Gladly, the book names the specific essential oils relevant in the creation of a fall-like environment and gives you recipes that you can use to produce just the right oil blend. Even for those who have never made candles of their own, you will see easy-to-follow steps provided in this book, which you can use to create scented candles customized to your needs.

The oils have been in use for medicinal purposes for thousands of years throughout history to treat a variety of different diseases. With the recent popularity of aromatherapy, the interest in essential oils has revived in the last decades. New consumers are discovering the many benefits they have to offer them, and they are curious how they can use them in a safe manner.

Chapter 1: Overview of Aromatherapy and Essential Oils

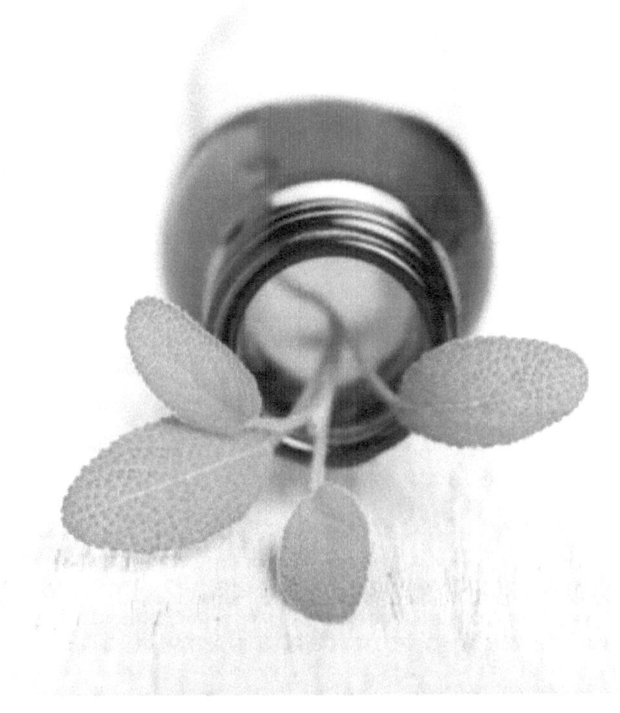

Essential oils are the essence of the herb, flower, or fruit rind. It is the most potent way to use herbals and other plant materials. They are made by either distilling the plant matter or pressing it.

Essential oils are safe, non-toxic, smell good, and are very effective in what they offer. These are just a few of the things that essential oils offer us. They are also very much at the center of aromatherapy (they are the mainstay ingredient in Aromatherapy blends and preparations), this is a wonderful way to improve both internal and external health through the use of fragrances that can help to evoke positive responses from us that in turn help to promote our health and well-being.

You will meet several essential oil blends to use. We will focus on recipes that offer the most benefits such as helping you to de-stress after a long and hard day at work. You need to relax and enjoy in the wonderful fall blends that will stimulate your external environment.

Using natural, holistic, and aromatherapy are great practices that are healthy and safe to use. The potential for them to help you in positive ways is limitless! You cannot put a price on the feelings of peace and contentment that you can achieve when you use essential oils in aromatherapy. With the use of essential oils you are able to treat all kinds of areas in your life including:

- stress
- asthma

- anxiety

- depression

- headaches

- stuffiness

- mood

- concentration

You can use the blends in this book to help to target that area in your life that needs that little extra boost. Decide on the blend or essential oils that will benefit you the most and the right diffuser to suit your needs. We will take a look into some wonderful recipes that will help to indulge your senses while offering endless benefits to you.

Essential oils are basically chemical substances with aromatic properties found in sources such as blossoms, seeds, bark, stalks, and other parts of plants. When using a diffuser to dispense your essential oils you want to make sure that you choose a diffuser that is suitable for your essential oils. Using a diffuser is a great way to freshen areas such as your work or home environment. I love using my diffuser as the final part of my house cleaning process. Once tidied, I then turn on my diffuser to give my home that fresh clean odor to match its fresh clean appearance.

Essential oils are not water-based photochemical made up of volatile organic compounds. Essential oils do not include fatty lipids as found in vegetable and animal oils but they are fat soluble. You will never experience an oily discomfort on your skin from essential oils in their pure form. Many cultures use essential oils as a form of healing benefits often they are dispersed through aromatherapy.

Cautions

There are several precautionary warnings that you should be well aware of when you are using essential oils.

- Certain essential oils such as lemon, ginger, clary sage, jasmine, chamomile, sage, cedarwood, and rosemary should not be used in your home if someone in your home is pregnant or nursing.

- It is always best to test your sensitivity to an essential oil before you use it. You can do this by simply combining one drop of essential oil with ½ teaspoon of olive oil. Rub this solution onto your arm and leave on for a few hours.

Check your arm regularly to look for signs of a rash or redness or perhaps even itching sensation that may be experienced in the region you applied the oil. If you find that you have had no reaction in several hours to the essential oil, then it means that you can safely use the oil.

- Make sure to keep your essential oils in a safe place just like you would any other medications in your household. They should be kept in places where kids cannot reach.

- Keep essential oils well away from your eyes as they could cause damage to your eyes.

- Do not take pure essential oil internally. Note that they are very highly concentrated forms and can be very potent indeed. You can add them with oils that you might buy at the supermarket to add to your foods. The oils that you buy at supermarkets are diluted for safe use.

- Do not overstock on your essential oils, most of them will last for about 5 years, and others may only last for 2 years. Keep in mind that you are only using a few drops of them at a time not the whole bottle.

- You do not aspire to use lots of money and buy too much essential oils that you will not use. It is always best to buy essential oils in small quantities.

- Do research on any essential oil that you are unfamiliar with. Make sure to do a test of it on your arm to make sure that you have no allergies to it. You will have over 100 different essential oils to choose from.

Following these simple tips and suggestions will help you to practice safe use of essential oils. The recipes that we are looking at in this collection are essential oil recipes for diffuser use.

Aromatherapy

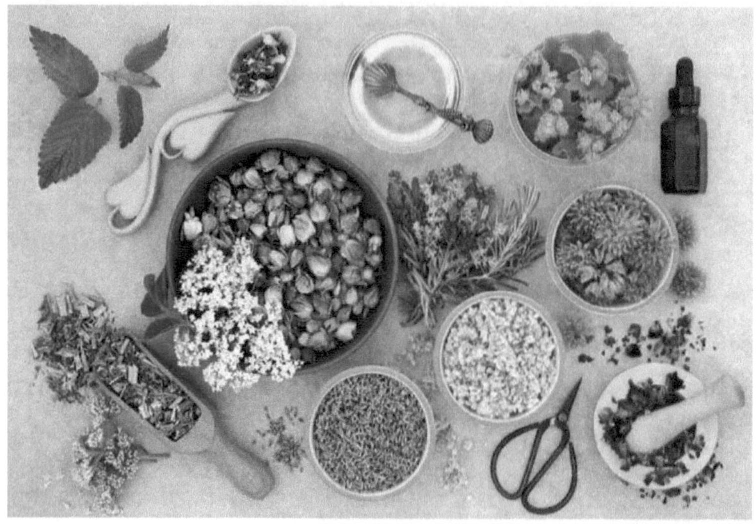

Aromatherapy is the act of using oils and scents to heal and enhance the body and mind. It is a practice that has spanned back thousands of years to the Ancient Egyptians, and still common in the present days.

Aromatherapy has a variety of applications, both physical and mental. Many people choose to use aromatherapy to achieve an overall sense of well-being, while others use it to aid in physical issues such as body aches and pains or immunity support.

Not only are the uses for Aromatherapy versatile, how you choose to administer aromatherapy is also varied. Common aromatherapy usage includes to diffuse essential oils into the air in various rooms of your house, but you can blend the oils with carrier oils and apply it directly to your skin, or you can add a few drops of these oils to your bath water and breathe deeply that way as well.

It doesn't matter too much how you administer your aromatherapy, but what does matter is how often you choose to partake in the therapy.

As with many natural remedies, you are going to see greater benefits if use it often, and let the benefits roll in over time.

Though several of the effects will be immediate (such as relief from a headache, feeling less tense or stressed, and sleeping better to name a few), other remedies make take a while before they kick in (depression and anxiety, for example).

When it comes to aromatherapy, you simply need to choose which method you would like to use as your primary and get started in that.

No worries if you are using essential oils in your bath water, or if you mix them and apply them directly to your skin is up to you, however, I strongly recommend that you also invest in a diffuser.

Diffusers are excellent options because they run for hours at a time, use minimal power, and can offer you benefits throughout your day, rather than you only being exposed to these benefits when you are actively trying to.

A diffuser in a corner of a room will send the warm therapy throughout the entire room, so if you place your diffuser well, you can expose yourself to the oils throughout the greater part of your day, which will increase the effectiveness of the benefits.

As you can see from the photos, there are a variety of diffusers you can choose from, so finding the look that goes with your décor isn't going to be an issue. You can go with something as bold or as subtle as you would like, fitting it into your day seamlessly.

The other thing to put into consideration is how long each diffuser is going to last on a single session. The different diffusers have different size tanks which last for set periods of time, depending on the diffuser you have chosen. A larger tank can last from 8 to 12 hours with constant use, while the smaller tank tend to last up to 2 hours.

Select the style based on your preference and your needs, and you are ready to get diffusing.

Can You Use Too Much Aromatherapy?

As with conventional medication, it's always wise to understand the risks and side effects of what you are doing, even for your health. When it comes to aromatherapy, whether you can overdose depends on your method of administration.

If you are diffusing your oils into the air, and you're also using the diffuser as it is intended to be used (in an open room, not intentionally concentrating the fumes for you to breathe in), then no, there is no chance of you overdosing on the oils.

Though the rich scents of each of the different oils is going to bring you healing, you aren't going to be exposed to a concentrated level that is enough to cause you any harm (when you are diffusing the oils).

However, if you choose to use the oils directly on your skin, you must be more careful. These oils are extremely powerful, and though they are made from entirely natural plants and roots, the concentration of each one has potentially harmful side effects if you use too much of it.

Thus, always mix your oils with another carrier oil before applying it to the skin, and why you are to follow scheduled administrations rather than constant exposure.

The most common side effect you are going to face with overexposure to these oils is skin irritation. Rash may occur, and in extreme cases, you may burn your skin. It is highly important that you use a carrier oil whenever you apply any of these oils directly to the skin, as the carrier oil will dilute the concentration enough that it won't cause irritation.

How Effective Is Aromatherapy?

First of all, aromatherapy has been practiced and observed for thousands of years. Even with the rise of modern medicine it has held its own among the rest, proving that there are dedicated followers who have gotten the results they were seeking.

When it comes to actual clinical trials, aromatherapy has proven to be incredibly effective, even more effective than conventional medication in some instances. Though when it comes to certain mental ailments such as depression conventional medication yields higher results, you don't have to face the same side effects, and you don't have to be careful to monitor how much of the oils you are using.

If you expose yourself to anxiety relief oils daily, you are going to find your anxiety subsides without having to worry about addiction or side effects. This is going to give you greater freedom to live your life as it was meant to be lived, without being held back by any condition.

When it comes to sleeping and an overall sense of well-being, essential oils have reigned supreme. Using your diffuser at night will not only put you to sleep faster, but it's going to help you stay asleep, resulting in more rest when you get up in the morning.

You will have greater clarity throughout your day, and a sharper sense of focus. Combined with the lack of anxiety and depression you feel, it won't be long before aromatherapy takes precedence in your life for all treatments and remedies you need.

Chapter 2: How to Use Essential Oils

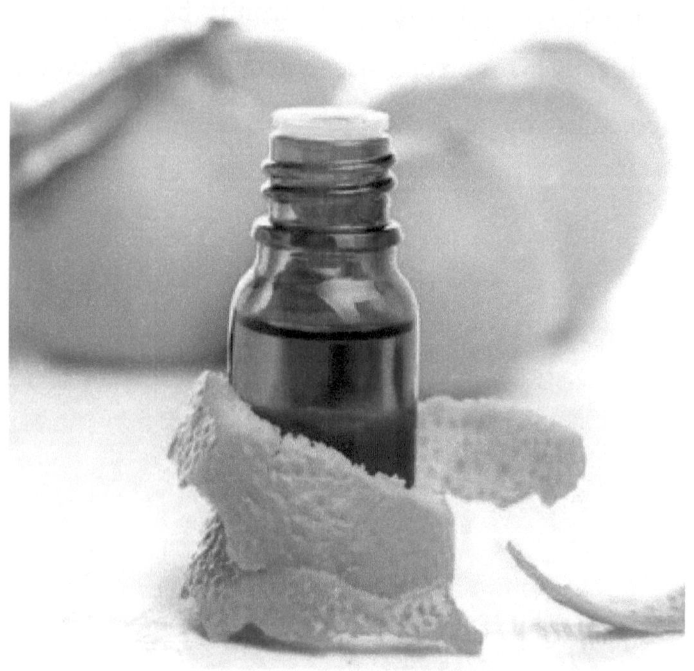

Essential oils have actually been in use since centuries ago, and even after many years of scientific medicine being used, people still want to explore the various uses they can put essential oils into. For one, it is gratifying to know that whether you are using the essential oil personally, or you are using them on your child, you are using something natural. It is rare that natural products cause you side effects, and so essential oils continue to be very popular even amongst the pharmacologically inclined folk.

Generations over the years have used essential oils extensively for aromatherapy, and people of diverse cultural backgrounds have been using them for their medicinal value. In fact, whereas essential oils were, for some time, not wholly embraced within the science fraternity, today scientists are exploring the possibility of deriving modern medicine from the same plants the essential oils come. As days go by, scientists maintain hope that one of these days they are going to discover a cure for stubborn ailments such as bronchitis, stroke, HIV, and many more.

There are three primary ways of using the essential oils:

Aromatically – Is my favorite way to affect mood and to open airways. Several oils can also be used aromatically to clean the air in your home.

Topically – Topical use of the essential oils can be extremely effective. Some people even say that an oil on you is an oil in you. A common place to use the oils topically is on the bottoms of the feet; this method of application will get you quick absorption into and circulation through the bloodstream.

Internally – Put them in your water, drop a single drop under your tongue, or fill an empty veggie capsule with a couple drops of the oils.

The other procedures of using aromatic essential oil include baths, massages, lotions, masks, inhalations, rinses, and aroma lamps. To avoid undesirable health effects, you should always consult a doctor before starting any aromatherapy.

Chapter 3: Flowers and Herbs to Use

Almond – Properties: Anti-inflammatory, protective

Argon - Properties: natural cosmetic, antioxidant phytochemicals, essential fatty acids, building brain capacity, digestive agent, blood sugar control.

Basil – Properties: antispasmodic, cold/fever reliever, digestive tonic, cough reliever, stress reliever.

Bay – Properties: antibiotics, antiseptic, Anti-Neuralgic, Anti-spasmodic, analgesic, sedative, stomachic and tonic.

Benzoin – Properties: sedative, relaxant, antidepressant, antiseptic, disinfectant, diuretic, anti-inflammatory, anti-rheumatic

Bergamot - Properties: Calming, hormonal support, antibacterial, antidepressant.

Black pepper - Properties: digestive, antispasmodic, aperient, Antirheumatic, Diaphoretic, antioxidant, antibacterial.

Black raspberry – Properties: antioxidants, anthocyanins, anticarcinogen, anti-viral, anti-bacterial, and anti-cancer properties.

Cajuput – Properties: antiseptic, Decongestant, Expectorant, analgesic, carminative, febrifuge, Antineuralgic.

Calendula – Properties: contains flavonoids and carotenoids, antimicrobial, antioxidants, anti-inflammatory, cell repair, Wound healing activity.

Camphor – Properties: Antiseptic, Disinfectant, Stimulant & Diaphoretic, carminative, anesthetic, antispasmodic, Antineuralgic, anti-inflammatory and decongestant.

Cedarwood – Properties: Anti-inflammatory, anti-fungal, antiseptic, antispasmodic, antidiuretic.

Chamomile – Properties: Sudorific, Febrifuge, Antiseptic, relaxant, anesthetic, Antibiotic, Disinfectant, Bactericidal, antidepressant, anti-inflammatory, stomachic, carminative.

Clary sage – Properties: Antidepressant, anticonvulsive, antispasmodic, antibacterial, antiseptic, carminative, euphoric, hypotensive, nervine, stomachic and digestive.

Clove - Properties: antitumoral, antimicrobial, antifungal, antiviral, analgesic, antioxidant, anticoagulant, anti-inflammatory, antiparasitic, stomach protectant (ulcers)

Coconut – Properties: Immunity, digestive, stress-reliever

Coriander – Properties: Aphrodisiac, lipolytic, carminative, antispasmodic, analgesic, depurative, stomachic, digestive, stimulant.

Cypress – Properties: anti-inflammatory, antiseptic, antioxidant, decongestant, sedative, styptic, mucolytic, hepatic.

Elemi – Properties: antiseptic, analgesic, expectorant, stimulant, and tonic.

Eucalyptus – Properties: anti-inflammatory, dental care, muscle pain, mental exhaustion, respiratory problems, wounds, intestinal germs, diabetes, fever, sauna, tuberculosis and pneumonia.

Fennel – Properties: antioxidants, antimicrobial, digestive, metabolism, circulation, antiseptic, antispasmodic, carminative, diuretic, laxative, stomachic, splenic and depurative.

Fir – Properties: respiratory support, antiseptic, pain reliever, detoxification, metabolism, respiratory agent, antibacterial, and antimicrobial.

Frankincense – Properties: stress reliever, digestive, anti-inflammatory, immune-enhancing abilities, anti-anxiety, astringent.

Geranium – Properties: dental health, anti-inflammatory, circulation, anti-stress, astringent, antibacterial, antimicrobial, hemostatic, cytophylactic, diuretic, styptic, and vermifuge.

Ginger – Properties: digestive, anti-inflammatory, anesthetic, antioxidants, anti-anxiety, menstruation, stomachic, anticoagulant, liver functioning, respiratory support.

Grape seed – Properties: immunity support, cancer prevention, wound healing, tonic and digestive.

Helichrysum - Properties: Anticoagulant, anesthetic, anti-inflammatory, antispasmodic, antiviral, liver protectant/detoxifier, regenerates nerves

Hyssop – Properties: astringent, antispasmodic, anti-rheumatic, antiseptic, digestive, diuretic, emmenagogue, expectorant, febrifuge, sudorific, vulnerary.

Jasmine - Properties: Uplifting, antidepressant, stimulating

Jojoba – Properties: anti-ageing, hormonal balance, anti-inflammatory, antifungal.

Juniper berry - Properties: Antiseptic, digestive cleanser/stimulant, purifying, detoxifying, diuretic, increases circulation through kidneys and promotes excretion of toxins, promotes nerve regeneration.

Laurel – Properties: antiseptic, antibiotic, anti-neuralgic, anti-spasmodic, astringent, cholagogue, febrifuge, sedative, stomachic, sudorific.

Lavender: Properties: Therapeutic effects, anti-inflammatory, first aid formula.

Lemon – Properties: immunity support, stomachic, digestive, bad breath remedy.

Lime – Properties: antiseptic, antiviral, astringent, febrifuge, haemostatic, restorative.

Mandarin – Properties: antiseptic, antispasmodic, circulatory, depurative, digestive, hepatic, nervous relaxant, cytophylactic, sedative and stomachic.

Marjoram – Properties: analgesic, antispasmodic, antiseptic, antiviral, carminative, cephalic, diaphoretic, digestive, diuretic, expectorant, vulnerary, laxative, stomachic.

Melissa – Properties: antidepressant, nervine, cordial, sedative, stomachic, carminative, sudorific, febrifuge, hypotensive.

Myrrh – Properties: antiviral, antimicrobial, astringent, expectorant, antifungal, carminative, stomachic, vulnerary, antiseptic, immunity support, anti-inflammatory, circulatory.

Neroli – Properties: antidepressant, antiseptic, carminative, antibacterial, disinfectant, sedative, digestive.

Orange - Properties: Antitumoral, relaxant

Oregano – properties: antioxidants

Palmarosa – Properties: antiviral, febrifuge, digestive, antiseptic, hydrating, cytophylactic.

Patchouli – Properties: antidepressant, antiseptic, astringent, cytophylactic, diuretic, febrifuge, sedative.

Peppermint – Properties: digestive, dental care, sedative, respiratory, immunity support, circulation, antimicrobial.

Pomegranate – Properties: immunity support, anti-inflammatory, circulation, stomachic.

Primrose – Properties: hormonal balance, fertility, anti-inflammatory.

Ravensara – Properties: analgesic, antimicrobial, antibacterial, antidepressant, antifungal, antiseptic, antiviral, diuretic, expectorant, relaxant.

Rose: Properties: Anti-inflammatory, antibacterial, antiseptic, laxative, anti-ageing properties, hydration, nourishment, heart comfort, mind stabilization/mental health, aphrodisiac, rejuvenation and toning.

Rosemary - Properties: Anti-inflammatory, relaxant, hydrating, skin-toning, reduces scarring, hormone balancing

Rosewood – Properties: antidepressant, analgesic, cephalic, antiseptic.

Sandalwood – Properties: anti-inflammatory, antiseptic, astringent, carminative, expectorant, diuretic, hypotensive, sedative.

Sesame – Properties: sedative, heart health, circulatory properties, metabolism booster, anti-inflammatory

Spearmint – **Properties:** antiseptic, antispasmodic, carminative, cephalic, restorative, emmenagogue.

Sunflower – **Properties:** immunity support, anti-inflammatory, energy enrichment, heart health.

Tea tree – **Properties:** antibacterial, respiratory effects, antifungal, antimicrobial, balsamic, antiviral, antiseptic, expectorant, sudorific.

Thieves – **Properties:** digestive, immunity support, respiratory health, anti-inflammatory.

Thyme – **Properties:** circulation, antirheumatic, antispasmodic, carminative, diuretic, expectorant, detoxification, sedative, vermifuge.

Turmeric- **Properties:** circulation, anti-inflammatory, detoxification, immunity support, antioxidants, stomachic.

Vetiver – **Properties:** antiseptic, nervine, vulnerary, anti-inflammatory.

Wheat germ – **Properties:** anti-inflammatory, heart health, antioxidants, metabolism booster.

Wintergreen – **Properties:** analgesic, anodyne, antirheumatic, antispasmodic, astringent, antiseptic, carminative, diuretic, emmenagogue.

Ylang ylang – **Properties:** antidepressant, antiseptic, hypotensive, sedative, nervine.

Chapter 4: Essential Oil Health and Healing Recipes

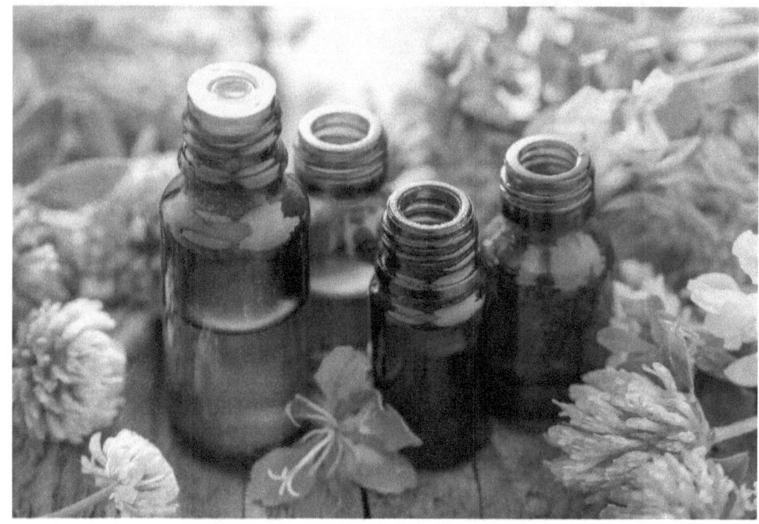

Here are some wonderful recipes to get you started on the path to essential oils. Try them all and mix your own blends. There's no end to the ways you can use these recipes through the seasons, regardless of summer or winter. Get ready to take your essential scents to a whole new level and enjoy the benefits of the seasons. You will fall in love with the scents – and the results – in no time.

Abdominal Pain

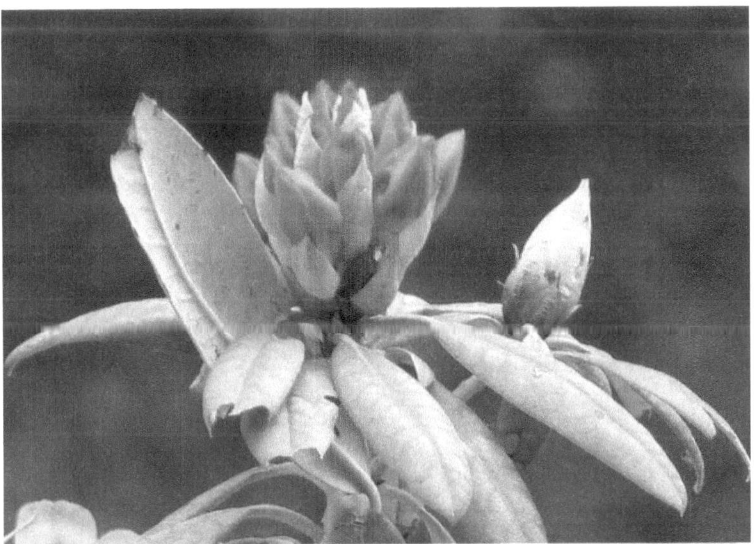

Abdominal pain is a common complaint which people make about and there are many reasons behind this pain however the most common reasons are

- Cystitis can result in abdominal pain
- Menstruation can cause abdominal pain
- Certain digestive problems can also cause abdominal pain
- Common muscle pulls also can cause abdominal pains

The best way through which abdominal pain can be treated is through Oil Massage and prescription for which is as follows

- About 5 Ml of carrier oil should be mixed with
- 1 drop of Peppermint oil
- 1 drop of calendula oil
- 1 drop of clove oil

Mix the above ingredients together and treat the area of the stomach with a gentle Massage. Clockwise fashion is advisable for the Massage.

Aches and Pains

Aches and pains can be as a result of various factors. Pain and aches may be a signal of disease, injury or illness which may interfere with your everyday activities. Such factors that may cause pain and aches include age, sprains, pitched nerves, arthritis, tendonitis, fibromyalgia, sprains, and neuralgia.

Recipe 1: Super Pain Reliever

Ingredients:

Essential Oils:

- 2 Drops Melissa oil
- 2 Drops Sweet Marjoram oil
- 2 Drops Chamomile oil

Carrier Oils:

- 10ml Carrier oil of your choice
- 10ml Jojoba oil

Preparation:

Blend all ingredients together and massage into affected areas twice daily or as needed.

You can also cut out the carrier oil and Jojoba oil and use these oils in a hot bath instead. If you are not epileptic and do not have high blood pressure, you can also add 2 cups of Epsom Salts and a half a cup of baking soda to the bath to help relieve pain.

Allergies

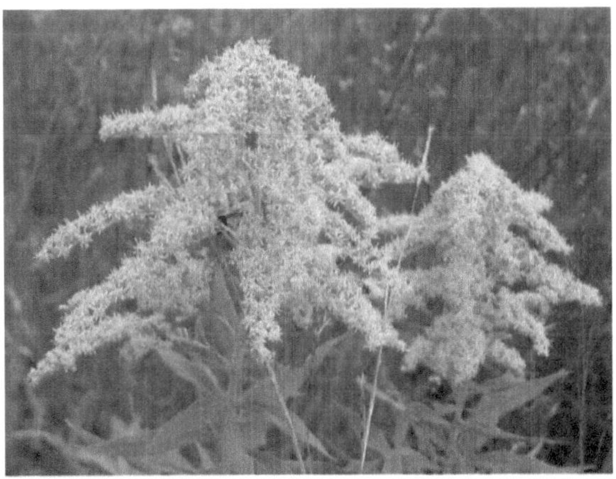

Many people around the world have developed an allergic reaction to different substances or allergens like food, pollen, tiny invisible particles, dust and pet dander. They always desire to get an effective solution to as an allergy reliever.

Recipe 1: Allergy Relief Recipe

Ingredients:

- 3 Drops of Eucalyptus Oil
- 2 Drops of Sandalwood Oil
- 2 Drops of Rosemary Oil
- 1 Blank Inhaler

Preparation:

Add all your ingredients to your blank inhaler and use inhaler whenever struck with allergy or hay fever attack.

Anal Fissures

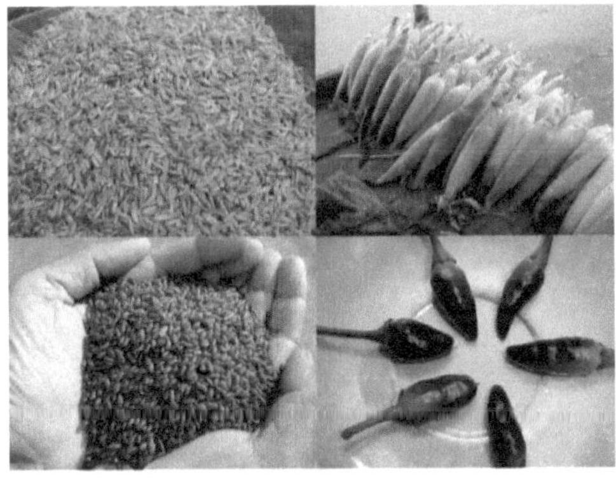

Anal Fissures can cause some serious pain and the prime reason behind Anal Fissures is Anal Disorders. The pain is usually accompanied with itching and happens during the movement of Bowels. The pain can happen to both children as well as adults.

Essential Oil treatment Recipe

Ingredients:

- Warm water
- 1 drop of lemon oil
- 5 drops of lavender oil

Preparation:

Get some warm water and place in a glass jar.

Add the essential oils to the water

Wash the affected area with this water

Anti-Ageing

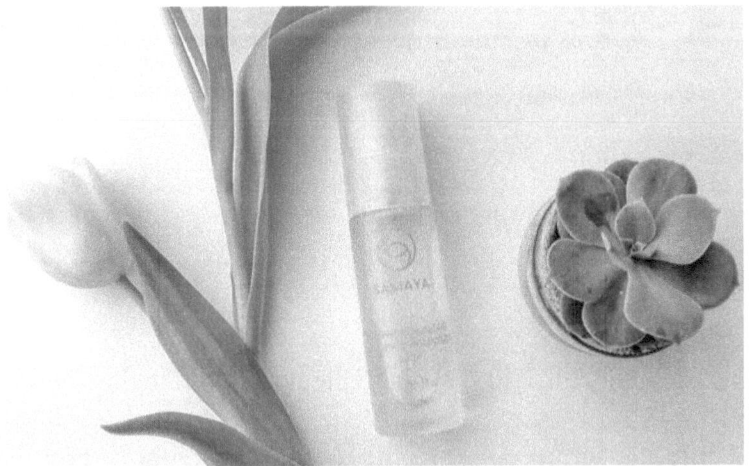

With the addition of years, the reality of ageing becomes real. Your body starts to weaken, your face starts to lose the glittering appearance it had and your joints become unsupportive. Essential oils can revert such cases.

Recipe 1: Cypress firming & Anti-Ageing serum

Ingredients:

- 2 tbsps. Rosehip seed oil
- 4 drops of Frankincense Essential Oil
- 7 drops of Geranium essential oil
- 7 drops of Cypress essential oil
- 2 tbsps. Sweet Almond Oil

Preparation:

Mix together all the above ingredients in a small glass bottle.

Apply the serum either in the morning or night or both as may be convenient.

Anti-Inflammatory Effects

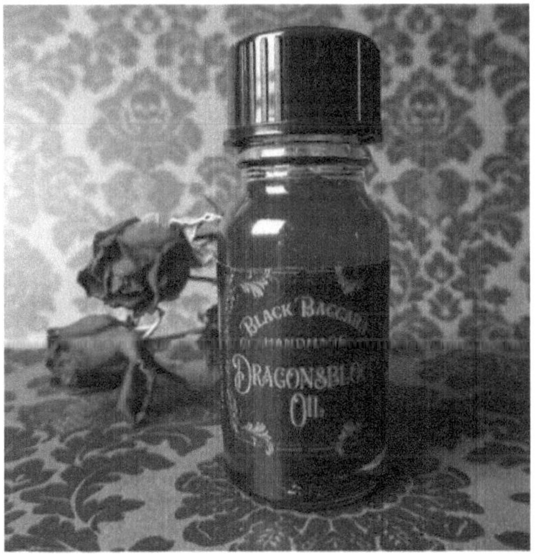

Recipe 1: The Frankincense blend

The Frankincense essential oil is the one you sometimes hear referred to as olibanum. It is a very unique type of oil that is extracted from a plant that requires very little soil to thrive. This oil that is very famous from the Christian Holy Book, the Bible, has a significant presence in Somalia, a country whose land is not particularly arable.

- Suggested ingredients:
- Frankincense essential oil – 5 drops
- Rose essential oil – 2 drops
- Hyssop essential oil – 3 drops
- Sesame oil – 2 drops

The Frankincense blend has antidepressant properties, and it is great for brain health. It also has anti-inflammatory properties. In addition, you can use it to relieve pain, and to eradicate external scars and wrinkles. It is also effective at preparing you for meditation, and you can bank on it to give you some grounding.

Anxiety

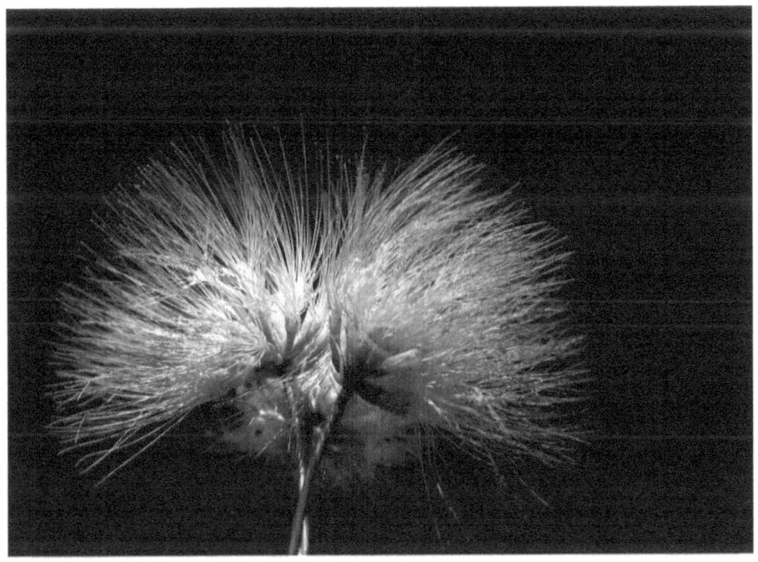

Recipe 1: Best Destress Ever!

If you have had a rough day, settle into this relaxing, anti-anxiety blend. You will want to stay forever.

Ingredients:

- ¼ cup of sunflower oil
- 8 Drops of Rosewood essential oil
- 2 Drops of Lavender essential oil

Preparation:

Mix ingredients and place in hot tub.

Appetite

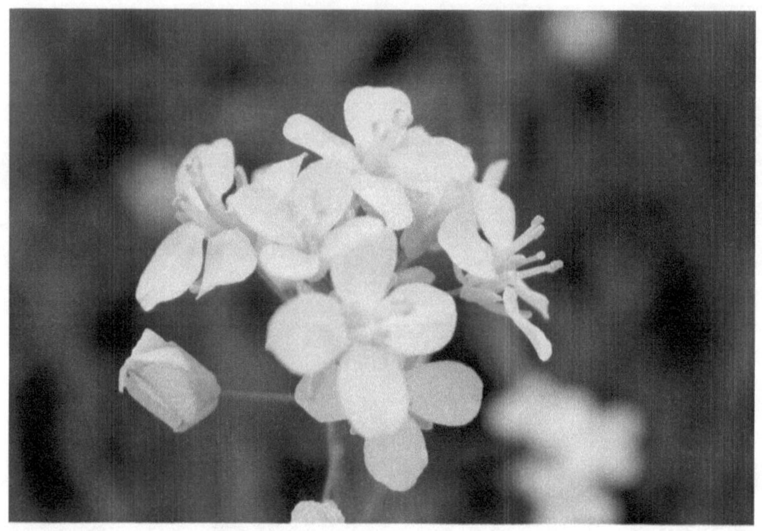

Recipe 1: Appetite Stimulant Recipe

Ingredients:

- 3 Drops of Lime Oil
- 3 Drops of Spearmint Oil
- 2 Drops of Ginger Oil

Preparation:

Mix all the ingredients together. Inhale directly from the bottle. Keep away from your eyes.

Arthritis

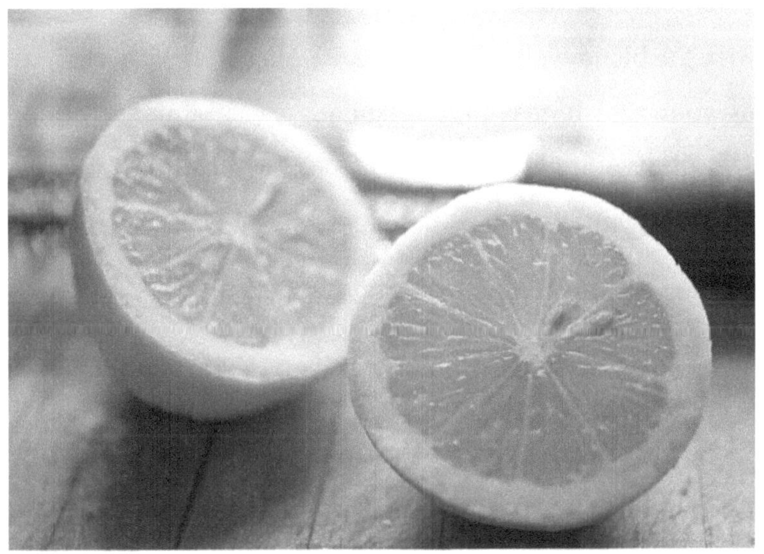

Recipe 1: Arthritis Eraser

Ingredients:

- 12 drops grapefruit oil
- 10 drops lemon oil

Preparation:

Direct Application Directions:

Mix the blend well, and if you are going to apply it directly to your skin mix with 2 teaspoons sweet almond oil and spread over the affected area. You may also mix with the lotion of your choice–do not ingest the oils.

Repeat every couple hours, or as often as needed.

Diffuser Directions:

Fill your diffuser with water as directed on the packaging, then add a few drops of this blend, also according to the packaging. Plug in your diffuser and place it where you will be able to sit or sleep nearby and breathe in the mist.

Continue to mist as needed.

Athlete's Foot

Athlete's foot is a very normal issue which people face particular those who are more involved in sports. Athlete's foot can cause itching and burning on the affected area.

The Treatment recipe

Make a mixture of 2 drops of wheat germ oil, 2 drops of tea tree oil, 2 drops of Geranium Oil and 10 ml carrier oil. Apply the solution gently around the nails and amid the toes. The treatment should be done every day.

Bedsores/Pressure Sores

The sores are caused by irritation and constant pressures. The bedsores can be painful.

Their Treatment Recipe

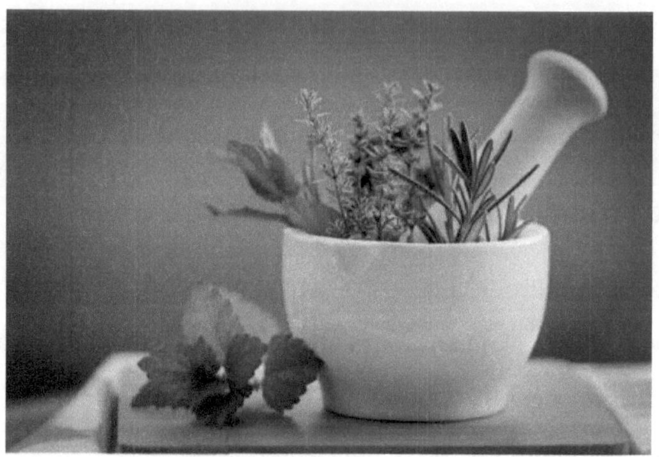

Ingredients:

- Massage oil has to be utilized

- 20 ml carrier oil

- 2 drops each of Frankincense oil, Lavender oil and Tea tree oil

- 4 drops of Wheat germ oil

- 3 drops of Geranium oil

Preparation:

The mentioned ingredients have to be mixed and the solution has to be applied on the affected areas.

In case of weeping bedsores, Massage Oil must not be applied

Bleeding Gums

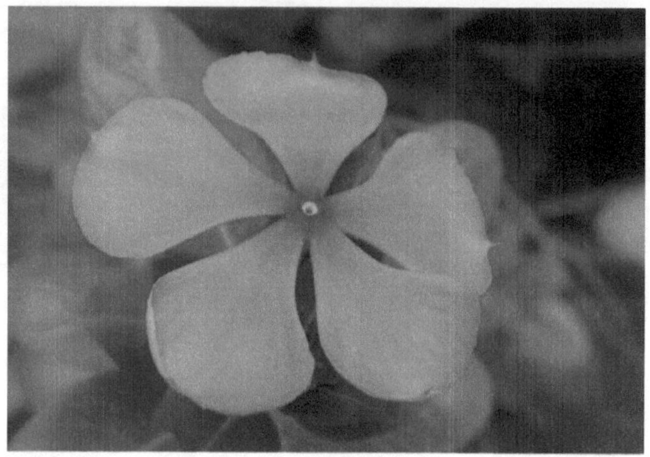

The main cause of Bleeding Gums is an infection known as gingivitis. The infection causes inflammation of the Gum.

The treatment recipe:

Develop a mouth wash

Add 3 drops of Thyme oil, Peppermint oil and Chamomile oil

Add Eucalyptus oil worth 2 drops

Do not swallow the mixture as it can cause adverse effects on health

Blisters

Blisters usually result due to some kind of burning, chafing and even insect sting.

The Treatment recipe is

- Apply the Lavender oil and Chamomile oil (1 drop each) on the affected portion

Blood circulation

The common sign of bad circulation is dizziness, fatigue, cold hands and high blood pressure etc. The essential oil treatment recipe for circulation issue is

- Prepare a Massage Oil having 2 drops each of Cypress essential oil, carrier oil, Neroli essential oil, Lemon essential oil and Geranium essential oil.
- Also add base carrier oil worth 15 ml

Boils

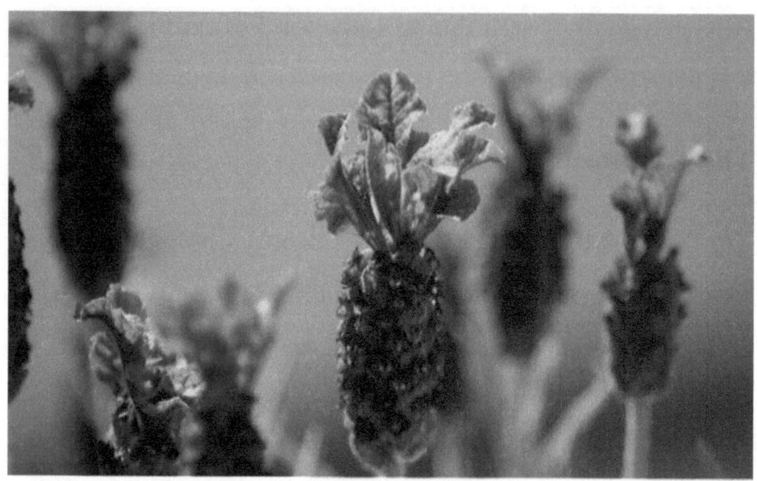

It is a kind of an abscess however as opposed to a normal abscess; Boils can cause Fatigue and Fever as well.

The Treatment Recipe is Ingredients:

- 200ml hot water
- 2 drops of lavender oil
- 1 drop of juniper oil
- 2 drops of tea tree oil

Preparation:

Place hot water in a container

Add the three oils to the water and mix

Wash the infected part of the body with this hot water

Bronchitis

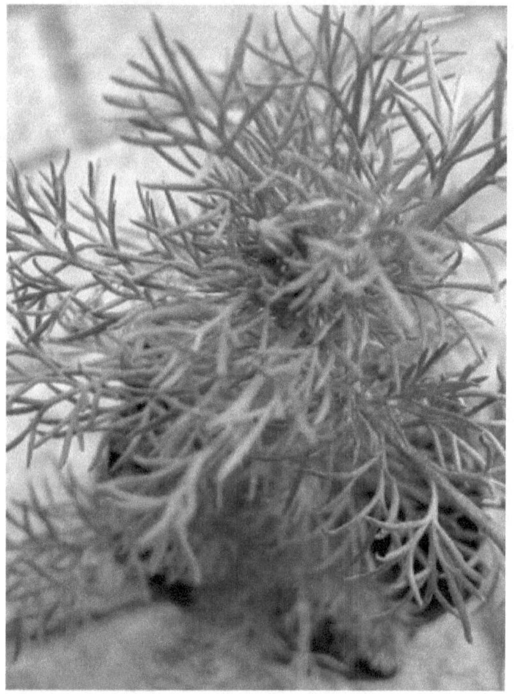

The cause of Bronchitis is cold and it is kind of infection which occurs on the bronchial tubes.

The Treatment recipe is

Inhalation therapy is

the best solution for Bronchitis

Essential oils such as Tea Tree oil, Basil, Pine, Benzoin and clove etc. can be used for Inhalation Therapy

Bruises

From the blood vessels which are damaged, blood escapes to other tissues which are under the skin causing Bruising.

The Treatment Recipe is

- Massage Oil should be utilized
- Cypress Oil worth 1 drop
- Calendula oil worth 5 drops
- Fennel oil worth 2 drops

All the mentioned oils should be mixed in 10 ml of Grape seed oil

Burns

Burns are usually measured in three degrees. If the burn is of first degree then redness will be seen. In case of second blisters will be visible and in case of third skin plus muscles will get damaged.

- Essential oils like Lavender can be utilized in case of minor burns. A damp compress can be used in this regard to cover the burned area
- For other kinds of burns professional advice is required

Colds, Flu and Congestion

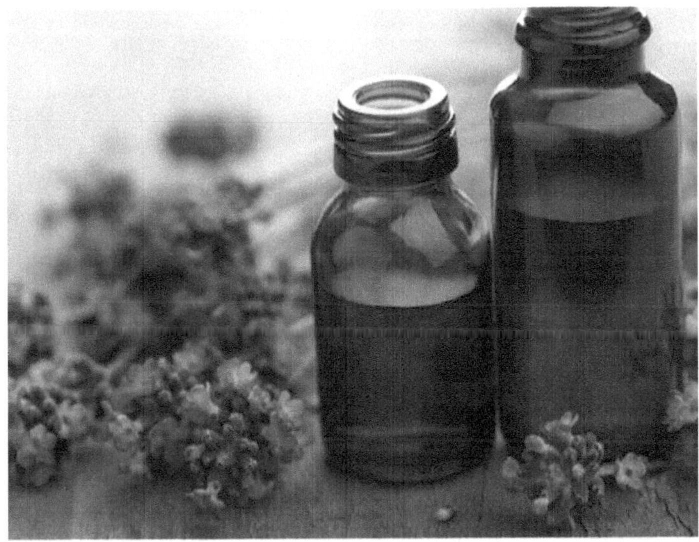

Colds are very common and can really make the human body lazy and lousy. Through essential oils flu and colds can be treated effectively by the following recipe

- 1 drop each of essential oils like Cinnamon, Pine, Cloves, Eucalyptus and Niaouli (this is more of a prevention measure)
- Oils like Cajuput, Pine, Niaouli and cloves can be utilized to treat stuffiness of cold
- The oils can be used through inhaler and can also be rubbed on the chest via bathing

Cold Sores

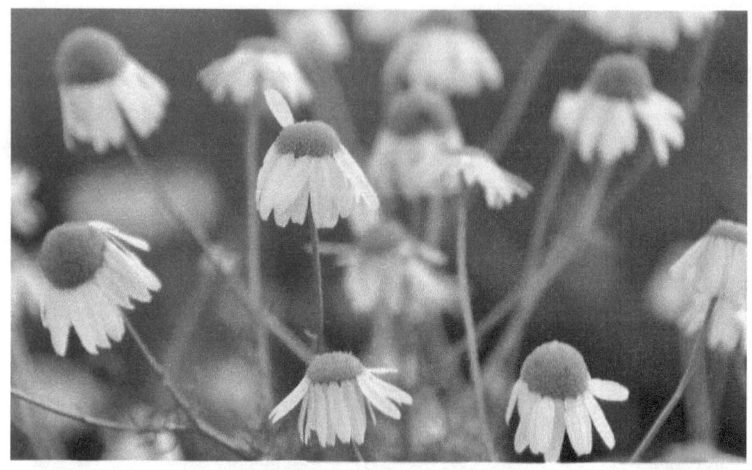

Sometimes blisters of painful nature appear around the lips. These blisters are known as cold sores. The treatment recipe related to cold sores is

- In order get rid of the pain use any of the mentioned oils
- Chamomile oil
- Geranium essential oil
- Tea tree oil

Coming Back to Normal After Fainting Episodes

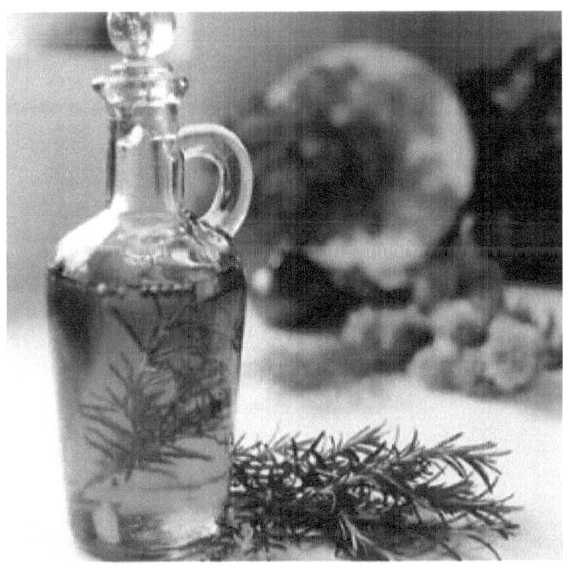

It usually happens due to the reduction of oxygen level in the brain and often results in consciousness's loss. The treatment recipe is

- Utilize the Peppermint oil and Rosemary oil. Make the patient inhale the oil's vapors and this can be done via opening the oil under the nose of the patient

- Give a solution containing hot water, lemon oil (1 drop) and honey (a teaspoon) to the patient when he or she gains consciousness

Constipation

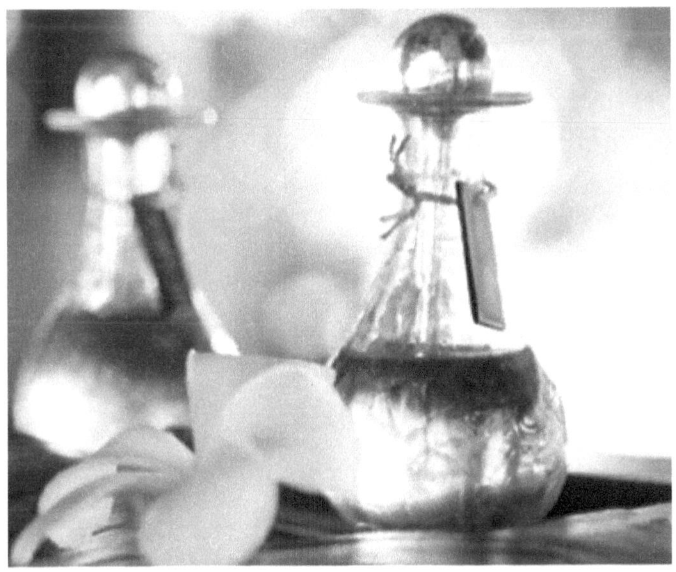

Constipation can be very irritating and it can make the normal procedures of body like passing of stools hard and painful. The treatment recipe is

- Prepare a Massage Oil having ingredients like
- Peppermint oil (5 drops), rosemary oil (15 drops) and lemon oil (10 drops)
- mix the mentioned oils in jojoba oil worth 30 ml
- Apply the massage oil three times a day on the lower abdomen. The Massage oil should be applied clockwise

Coughs

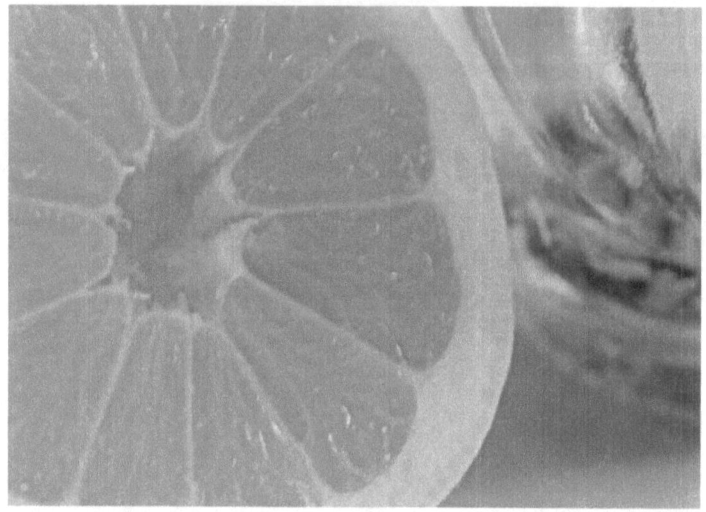

When the human body reacts to any irritation or disorder in the respiratory system then the resulting phenomenon is a cough. The treatment recipe of coughing is

Develop a mixture for drinking purpose

The mixture should contain 2 drops each of Lemon oil, Eucalyptus oil and 3 tablespoons of honey

Add 1 teaspoon of this mixture in water worth half a glass

Drink the mixture slowly

Dandruff

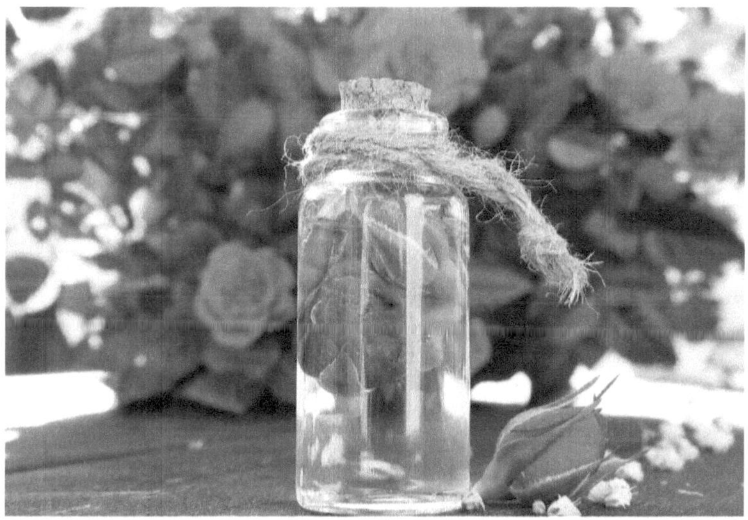

Don't look like you have been in a snowstorm if you haven't been.

You will need:

- ½ cup of jojoba oil
- 8 Drops of Rosemary essential oil
- 5 Drops of Tea Tree essential oil

Mix the ingredients together and apply to head. Let sit for 10 minutes. Rinse.

Dental Problems

When teeth hurt, your entire body hurts. You may have an infected tooth or an abscess or a cavity that is growing more damaging. Leaving your infected tooth alone will cause swelling of the face, swollen lymph nodes, and a fever. If an abscess ruptures, it will leave a foul-tasting liquid in your mouth, and if left untreated it will spread to other areas of your neck and jaw. Before you can get to the dentist, you might want to use clove oil, helichrysum, tea tree oil, frankincense, chamomile or wintergreen on the abscess. Use any of these or a mixture of several as a compress and apply to the affected area. You can use clove or peppermint oil by applying one or two drops to a cotton ball and applying to the gums in the area of the toothache.

Depression

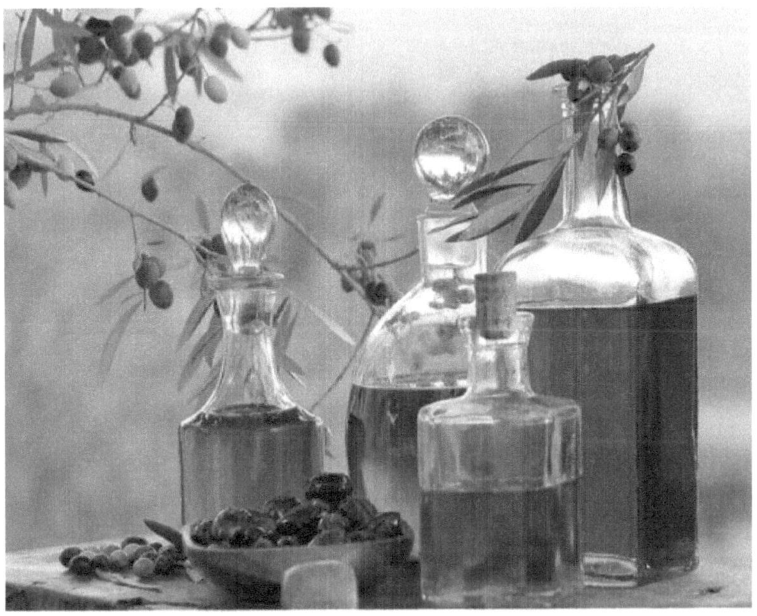

Lift depression the safe and effective way.

You will need:

- ¼ cup of olive oil
- 20 Drops of Frankincense essential oil
- 10 Drops of Lavender essential oil

Mix together and breathe in for a good period of time. Apply to chest and under your nose too!

Diarrhea

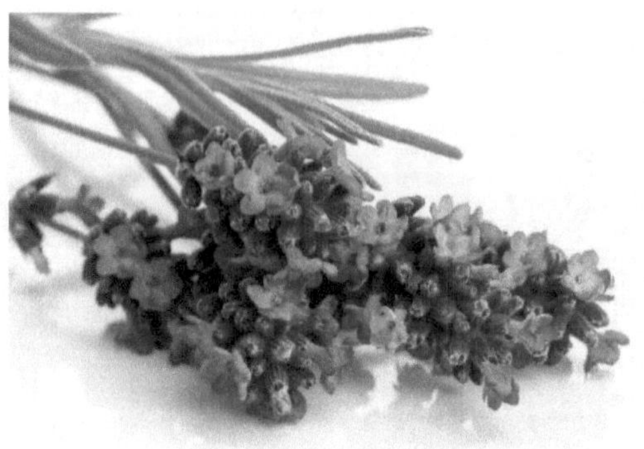

Diarrhea is a very painful disease and it is an indication that there is some kind of disorder in the bodily system. In case the mucus membranes get inflamed then fever can also happen to the patient. The treatment recipe is

- Add 2 drops each of Peppermint oil, Geranium oil, Chamomile oil, Lavender oil and Eucalyptus oil in 10 ml vegetable carrier oil to make a proper massage oil
- Rub the massage oil gently on the abdominal area for quick healing

Ear Infections/Earache/Ear-Related Ailments

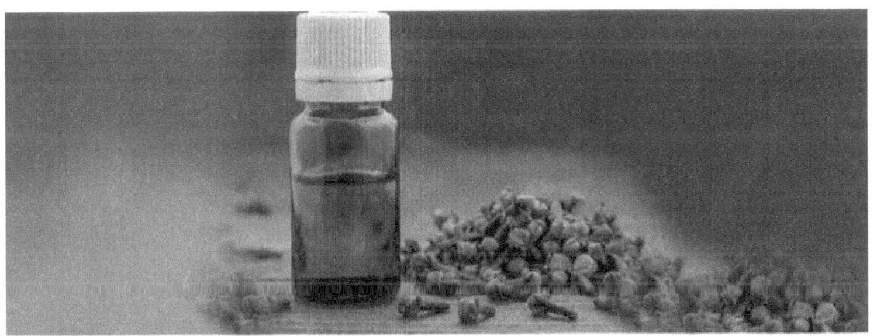

Middle ear function is the prime cause of Earache and its treatment recipe is

- Make a mixture of Grape seed oil (5ml) and Clove oil (1 drop)
- Use the solution by massaging the area around the ear and neck as it will cause reduction of pain

Eczema

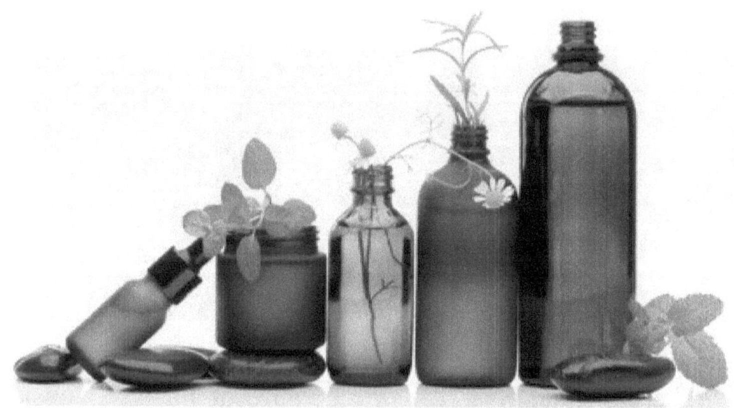

Eczema Cream Lotion

Ingredients:

- two tablespoons of beeswax
- 3 ounces of Shea butter
- 3 tablespoons of sweet almond oil
- 12 drops of vitamin E oil
- 12 drops of lavender essential oil
- 12 drops of German Chamomile essential oil

Directions:

In a double broiler melt your Shea butter and beeswax. Mix well. Allow for it to cool at room temperature. Add in the essential oils. Cool completely before using lotion.

Hiccups and Halitosis

Hiccups or the uncontrollable spasms of the diaphragm, caused by a sudden intake of breath and the closure of the glottis, can be debilitating. Something irritating the diaphragm or carbon dioxide in the bloodstream are possible causes of hiccups. They are annoying, can be painful and embarrassing. Get rid of hiccups by using sandalwood essential oil. You may directly inhale from the bottle or diffuse into the air. Apply the oil to hands, tissues or on a cotton ball and inhale.

High Blood Pressure/ Hypertension

Those ailing from hypertension or high blood pressure will benefit from using lemon, ylang-ylang, marjoram, eucalyptus, lavender, clove, clary sage, lemon, and wintergreen. You can add several drops of any of these oils in a bath to give you a stress relieving session and to lower your blood pressure. Mix five drops of geranium, eight drops of lemongrass oil, and three drops of lavender in a carrier oil like fractionated coconut oil. Gently rub over your heart and reflex points on the left foot and hand. Feel the stress melt away.

Insomnia

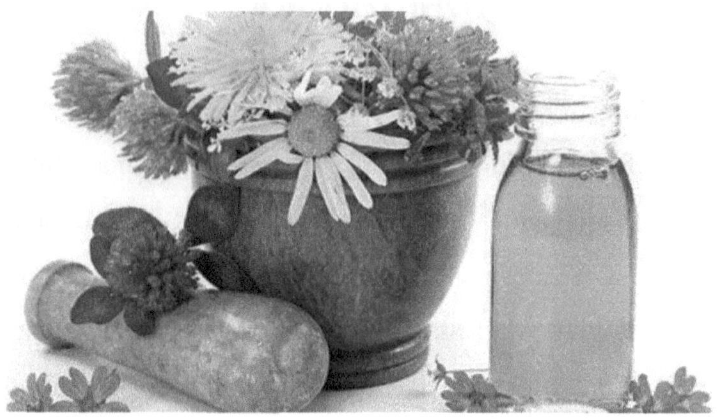

If face challenges to fall or to stay asleep, essential oils can be the answer for you. Stress, medications, drug or alcohol use, anxiety and depression are just some of the causes of insomnia. Combine 6 drops of orange with six drops of lavender. Apply this blend to big toes, and bottoms of your feet. Put a couple of drops around the navel and three drops on the back of the neck. You can also combine two drops of Roman chamomile, six drops of geranium, three drops of lemon, and four drops of sandalwood and a good carrier oil in a dark glass bottle. Shake to mix and add six drops of this mixture to your bath before bedtime. Add a little more power to your sleep and spray lavender essential oil on your pillow. Spraying lavender should do the trick and cure your insomnia.

Irritable Bowel Syndrome

Irritable bowel syndrome is a intestinal disorder characterized by diarrhea, gas, constipation, and bloating, cramping, and abdominal pain. It is a very common disorder and also very painful. You can feel much better if you add two drops of peppermint oil and two drops of Chamomile to eight ounces of distilled water and drink at least 1-2 times a day. You can also place two drops of these oils in an empty capsule and swallow. It will feel great to your sore and tired tummy if you dilute 1-2 drops in fractionated coconut oil and apply over the abdomen and then use a hot compress.

Itching & Hives

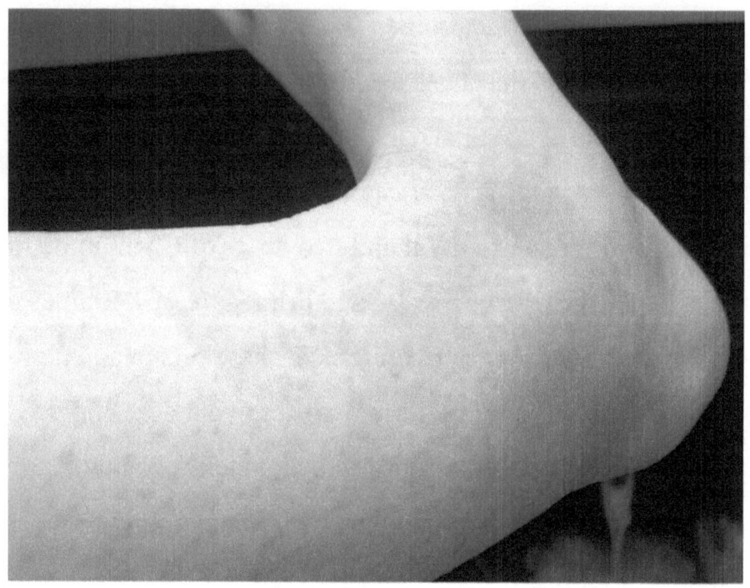

Itch Reliever Bath Salts

I love to use this in the winter when my skin is so dry and itchy—it really works wonders!

Ingredients:

- 1 c. sea salt
- 5 drops lavender essential oil
- 5 drops peppermint EO
- 5 drops Jasmine EO
- 2 tbsps. baking soda

Directions:

Mix the salt in a bowl with other ingredients. Add one drop of essential oil at a time as you continue to stir the mixture. Allow the mixture to dry for six hours store it in a glass jar.

Muscle/Joint Pain and Vitality

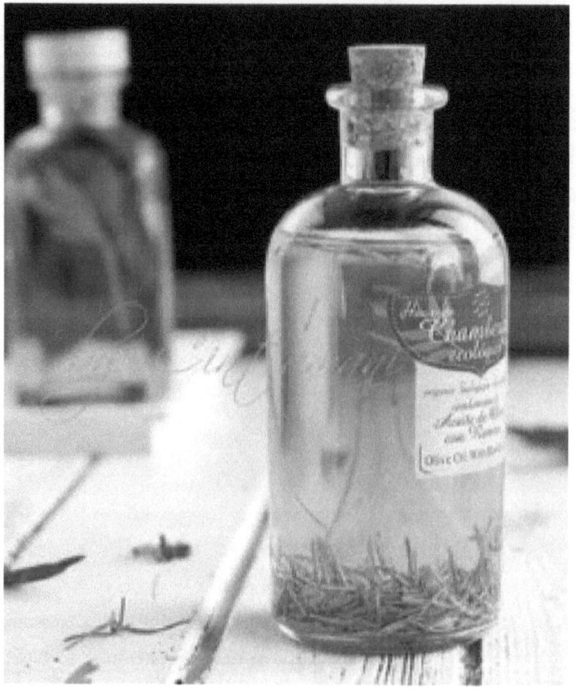

Your achy muscles will feel as good as new with this remedy.

You will need:

- ¼ cup of olive oil

- 20 Drops of Peppermint essential oil

Mix and apply to the source of pain.

Psoriasis

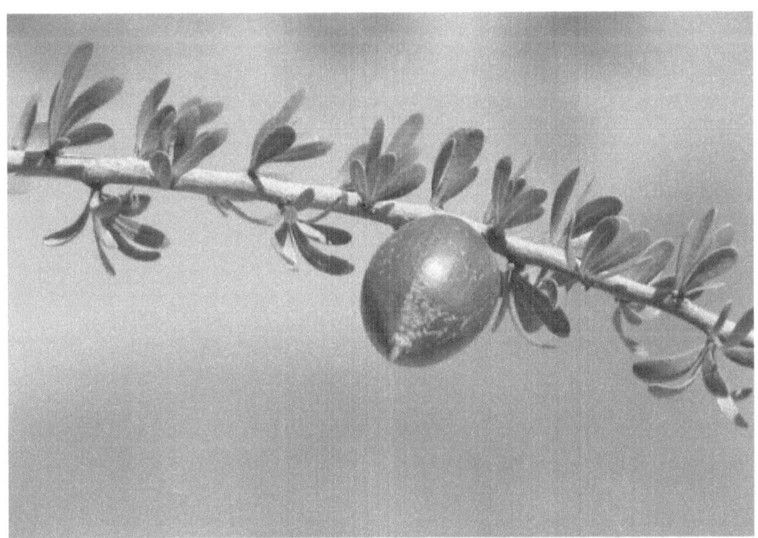

Psoriasis Body Oil

Ingredients:

- 5 oz. of apricot kernel oil

- 12 drops of Helichrysum essential oil

- 12 drops of Bergamot essential oil

- 2 oz. of pomegranate oil

Directions:

Mix your carrier oils and essential oils in dark glass bottle.
Shake well before each use.

Rash

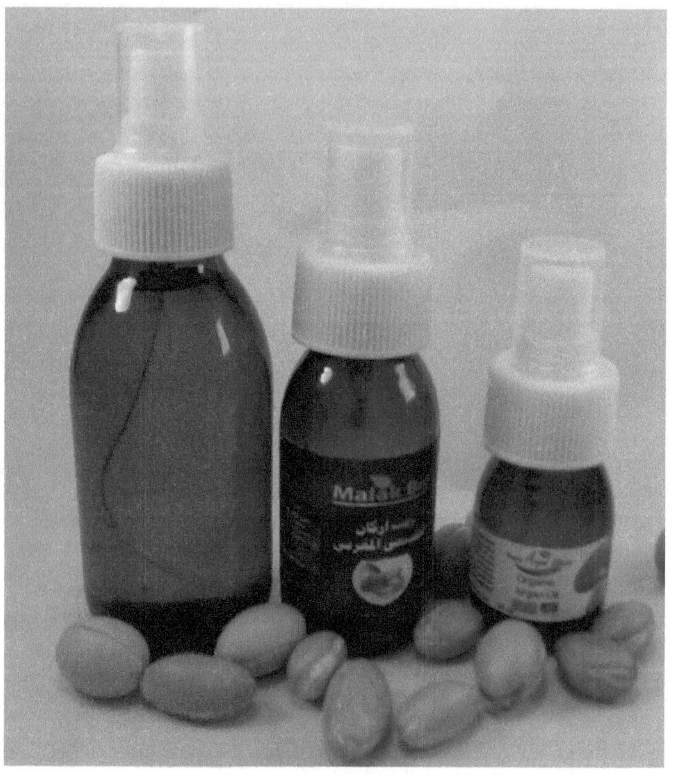

Works wonders to relieve rashes fast.

You will need:

- ½ cup of argon oil

- 20 Drops of Rosemary essential oil

- 5 Drops of Tea Tree essential oil

Mix and apply.

Teeth Whitener

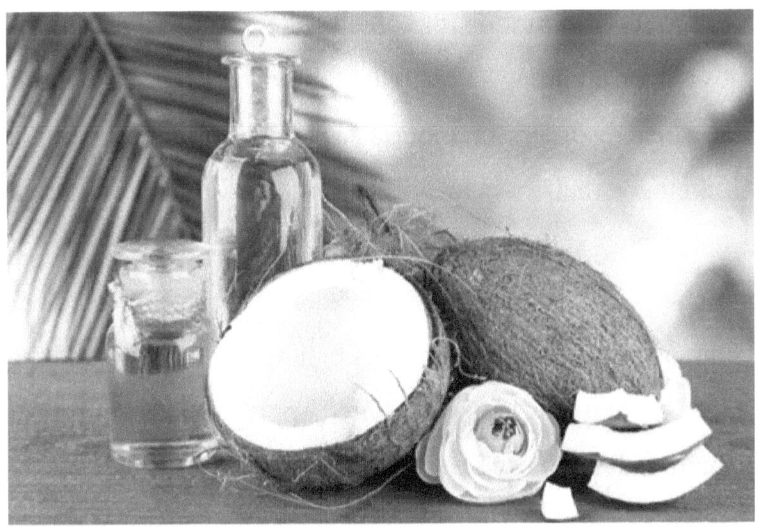

You will need:

- 10 Tablespoons of coconut oil
- 5 Drops of Lemon essential oil

Spread onto teeth with fingers and allow to sit for 10 minutes, then rinse.

Vertigo

Vertigo is a sensation that feels like the environment is moving or spinning. You may fall or feel nauseated. Ear infection, disorders or motion sickness can cause vertigo. Use ginger, helichrysum, geranium, basil and lavender to combat the symptoms of vertigo. Apply 1-2 drops of helichrysum, geranium, and lavender to the tops of each ear and massage it in. Apply the oils behind each ear, behind the jaw bone and just below the jaw. Apply 1-2 drops of basil behind and down each ear.

Wound Ointment and Dressings/Infected Wounds

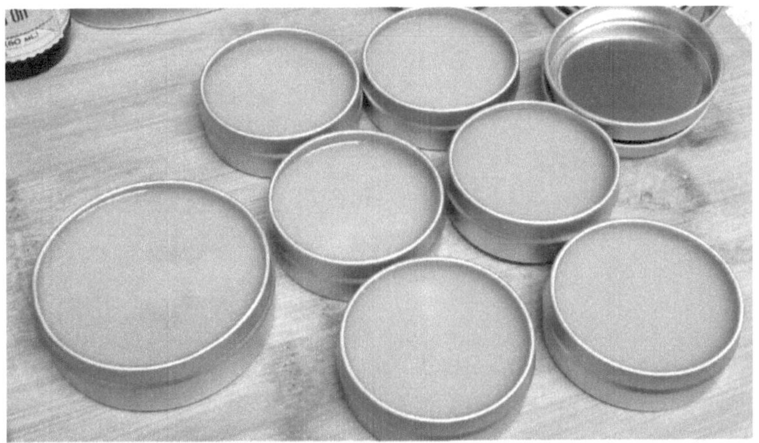

Wound care requires a few key anti-microbial essential oils. Number one on the list is melaleuca or tea tree oil. With its properties as an antiseptic and antimicrobial it is perfect for cleaning and dressing wounds. You can also dip into your stores of lavender if you are treating a wound. Lavender speeds up the healing process of wounds and improves the formation of scar tissue. It is also pain-relieving. Use helichrysum to keep your wounds from turning septic. Helichrysum is safe to apply on wounds, cuts, and pricks or any other open sores that are in danger of becoming infected. Helichrysum is also a coagulant that helps with bleeding.

Wrinkles

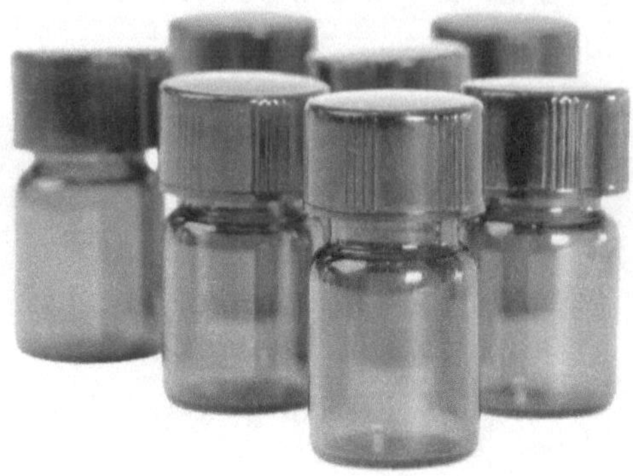

Wrinkle Prevention Serum

Ingredients:

- 2 drops of Lemon essential oil
- 2 drops of Rosemary essential oil
- 10 drops of Carrot essential oil
- 10 drops of Primrose essential oil
- 10 drops of Fennel essential oil
- 10 drops of Lavender essential oil
- 10 drops of Neroli essential oil
- 3 tablespoons of Almond oil

Directions:

Mix the carrier and essential oils together then store in dark glass bottle. Shake well before each use. Use two to three drops daily on face and neck.

Conclusion

Practice each recipe until you find your favorites, and experience life like you used to. Get out, have some fun, make those crafts, and be the person you used to be. Pain is no longer going to hold you back, so live like you mean it!

Enjoy the journey!

Author's Afterthoughts

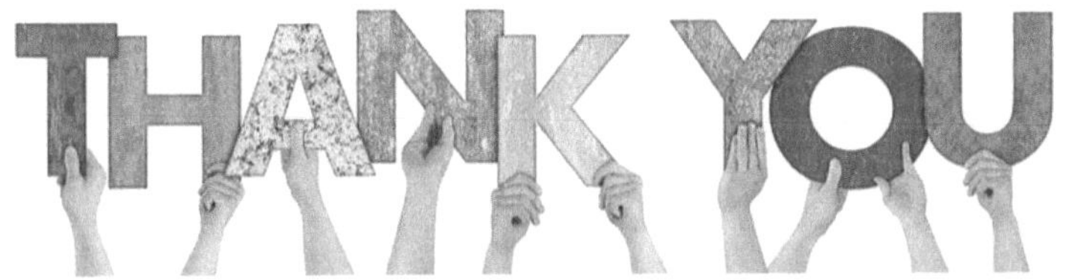

With so many books out there to choose from, I want to thank you for choosing this one and taking precious time out of your life to buy and read my work. Readers like you are the reason I take such passion in creating these books.

It is with gratitude and humility that I express how honored I am to become a part of your life and I hope that you take the same pleasure in reading this book as I did in writing it.

Can I ask one small favour? I ask that you write an honest and open review on Amazon of what you thought of the book. This will help other readers make an informed choice on whether to buy this book.

My sincerest thanks,

Angel Burns

If you want to be the first to know about news, new books, events and giveaways, subscribe to my newsletter by clicking the link below

https://angel-burns.gr8.com

or Scan QR-code